To My Dear Friend.
So Glad your in
my life.
Love Rita
You

Author's Note

When I was in high school, my grandfather was diagnosed with rampant Stage 3 cancer. He was told that it was too invasive to treat with surgery and he probably had just two more weeks to live. At best, he might survive two more months.

I remember the absolute determination in my grandfather's eyes as he declared, "I'm not going anywhere until I finish all the things I want to do! Give me the medicine!" With the help of my mother, he pushed through his chemotherapy and radiation treatments. Six months later, he refused the follow up therapies. He made a firm announcement, "It's done! I have other things to get back to now." Then he went about accomplishing all the goals he had set for himself.

After nearly two years, my grandfather completed his to-do list and his cancer came back full force. He surrendered to it and passed away without regret. Before he died, he gave me the thumbs-up and said, "You numbah one! Do your best!" Then he pointed to his temple saying, "Your mind strong. Make your life numbah one!" He was a powerful force to his very last day and he left an indelible mark in my life. He showed me how the power of our minds and spirits can affect our being.

I recognized that same thumbs-up attitude in every woman I interviewed for this book. Each of these courageous women is a shining example of spirit in action. While there are similarities, no two stories are the same, no two spirits identical. Each woman has her own unique recipe for survival. All of their stories are uplifting, powerful, touching and deserving of our admiration and respect. They are not simply "Survivors." They are thriving spirits, true examples of the power of passion, courage, faith and love. I am grateful to each and every one of them and I am deeply touched and honored by their willingness to show their souls to us.

I believe that we each possess a unique and powerful spirit and when we nurture it, we tap into a power greater than ourselves. In Hawai'i we have a simple greeting that is a powerful blessing. *"E Mālama Pono."* It means "Take care, stay well, be integrated with your mind, body, and soul and the world." My hope is that these stories and portraits will inspire you to recognize the unique spirit that lies within you. And prompt you to honor, feed, and nurture that very special part of you.

E Mālama Pono. May your spirit thrive.
~ Cynthia Y. H. Derosier

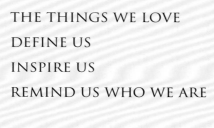

THE THINGS WE LOVE
DEFINE US
INSPIRE US
REMIND US WHO WE ARE

GIVE US STRENGTH
HELP US HEAL
CALM OUR GREATEST STORMS

THROUGH THEM
WE RE-CREATE
LIVE LIFE OUT
BREATHE LIFE IN
WE PRAY IN OUR OWN WAY

OUR BODIES RESPOND
REVELING IN
THE POWER, THE PASSION
AND BEAUTY OF OUR SOULS

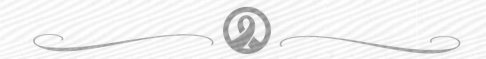

These are the songs of the Survivor Spirit...

Fear or faith?
I chose to be carried by absolute faith

I have always been a survivor. When I discovered the lump in my breast, I had already survived battery and spousal abuse as well as a drug addiction. Yet, of all the things I had to deal with up to that point, cancer was the one thing I knew I couldn't control.

Cancer isn't the kind of stuff you can sweep under the rug, cover up with makeup, or fix with a pill, drink or smoke. Even though you can't see it, it's there. You have to deal with it head on. My mother had died of cancer because she ignored it for years. When she finally went to the doctor, the tumor was the size of a cantaloupe and had spread everywhere. I was scared but I knew I couldn't ignore it.

I stayed focused in the moment, not letting the fear of the future get a hold of me. I stopped everything, prayed to God, and knew if I had any chance at all, it was to get myself to the doctor right away. Within hours of finding the lump, I was officially diagnosed with cancer. A week later I had a mastectomy. That was over 20 years ago.

I really started growing spiritually in my recovery. I had absolute faith that no matter what happened I would be able to deal with it and I had to take the next step on the path laid out in front of me. Just close my eyes, let go and believe in my higher power.

My tattoos are my badges of honor. Some of them are over my mastectomy and reconstruction scars. All of them are empowering reminders to me that through a leap of faith I made it through the battles and won the war of my life.

~ Claire McDaniel

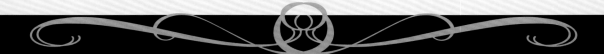

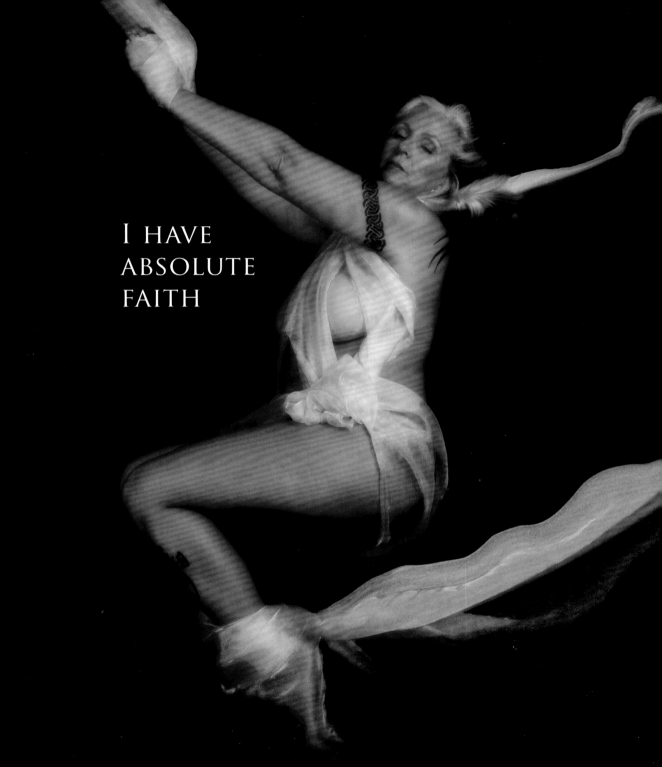

I HAVE
ABSOLUTE
FAITH

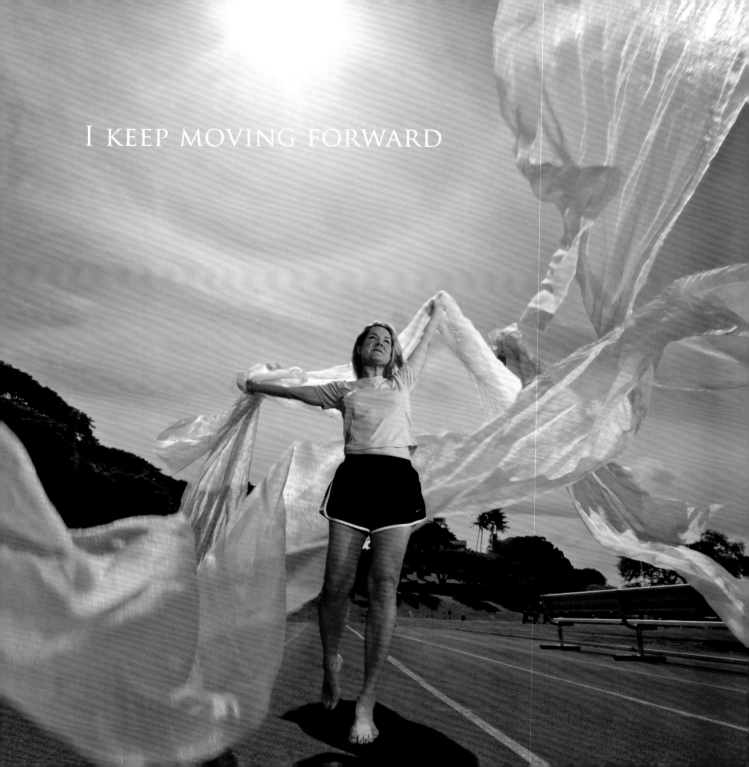

I KEEP MOVING FORWARD

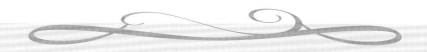

Running the race of my life

I've always been a jogger, nothing too heavy, just enough to stay in shape and have fun. I never thought breast cancer would happen to me. When we found three cancerous sites in my breasts I was devastated. I felt like time had run out. I bargained with God "Please just give me five years to watch my son grow." I thought of him and started fighting. I wanted everything. Whatever treatment I could have, I took.

My son is a runner and the thought of him kept me inspired. Fighting cancer is like running a race. You have a course of treatment with a certain number of markers and you have to do the entire course in order to win. No matter how much it hurts, you just keep moving forward. Just take the next step.

And like a race, it isn't always easy. No pain, no gain. There were days when my body was so fatigued I could barely move, forget about running, but I made myself get up and walk a little. Moving just a few steps always made me feel better in my mind, if not my body.

I've been in every Race For The Cure run including the ones before I had cancer. Since then, I've run my first marathon and raised $2,300 for the Leukemia Society. We all have to keep moving forward and keep giving back until we find a cure. Never stop. Never give up.

~ Suzanne Ditter

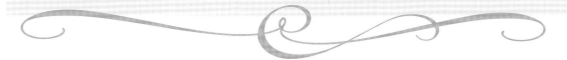

THE DREAMS AND TRADITIONS OF FAMILY
GIVE POWER TO OVERCOME

I am alive because of my family and friends. My father passed away when I was young and my mother raised me and my brothers. When I became ill, my brother offered to take care of me and help with my bills as if he were my dad. My future husband was always strong and committed to taking care of me too.

At first, my family was very worried when I had decided to go with Asian holistic treatment, *Kampo*, instead of western chemotherapy. We had many long conversations about my choice and my family was very uncomfortable with my commitment to it. But then, my mother had a dream that took away her worry and gave everyone confidence in my choice.

In my mother's dream, she saw me going into a dark hole that was full of snakes. She called out to me, "Emi, come back!" When I came out of the hole holding a turtle, my mother said "You are safe." In Japanese culture, dreams are thought to be messages from our ancestors. Turtles are said to live for a million years and are interpreted as a sign of longevity. My mother and I believe my father sent the dream to let us know that I had the power to overcome my cancer.

The dream reassured my mother and gave me more strength knowing that my father was protecting me. Today, I am healthy and happy and appreciate my family and friends more than ever. They have always takes care of me and I know I am safe.

~ EMI HANAMIZU

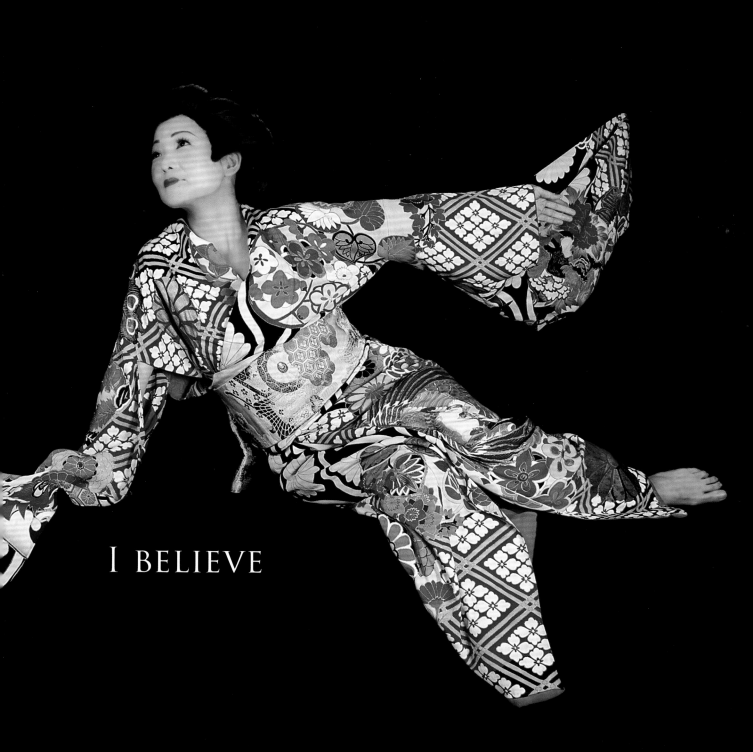

I BELIEVE

Prepared for heaven on earth
or heaven above

After my sister passed away from ovarian cancer, I got tested and found I have the same genetic profile. When I developed breast cancer, I felt a strange sense of calm. Because I had been with my sister through her illness, I felt totally prepared for the physical and emotional challenges ahead. I didn't want to leave my family, but if I didn't survive I wanted to make the most of my time and do everything I could to make things easier for those I left behind.

When I was ill during treatments, my children gave me strength. One day my two youngest asked what was wrong. I told them, "Some people get cancer. It gets in their blood and makes things go wrong and makes things grow. Some people need medicine, and they get sicker before they get better. And some people, medicine can't help. God has a special job for everyone, but we don't know his plans for me. He might have more work for me here or he might need me in heaven."

Either way, I assured them I'd be nearby. I put my hands over their hearts and put their hands over my heart. I told them, "We'll always be together in our hearts." If God needed me in heaven, someone else would be here for them and they'd be okay. Then we talked about what an awesome place heaven is.

We made a deal: if I got to heaven first, I would get our house in heaven ready. I'd have a pasture with a herd of horses for my daughter. I'd get my son a strong bed because he knew animals in heaven are gentle and he wanted to sleep with a pet lion. It helped them to know I would be in a good place, and we would be together again in heaven some day.

Since ovarian cancer and breast cancer are linked to the same genetic defect, I had a full hysterectomy and a double mastectomy. I don't know if I'll get cancer again or how long I'll be around, but I'm grateful for every moment I have here and when God needs me up there, I'm cool with that, too. I have faith in God's plans.

~ Brenda Schroeder

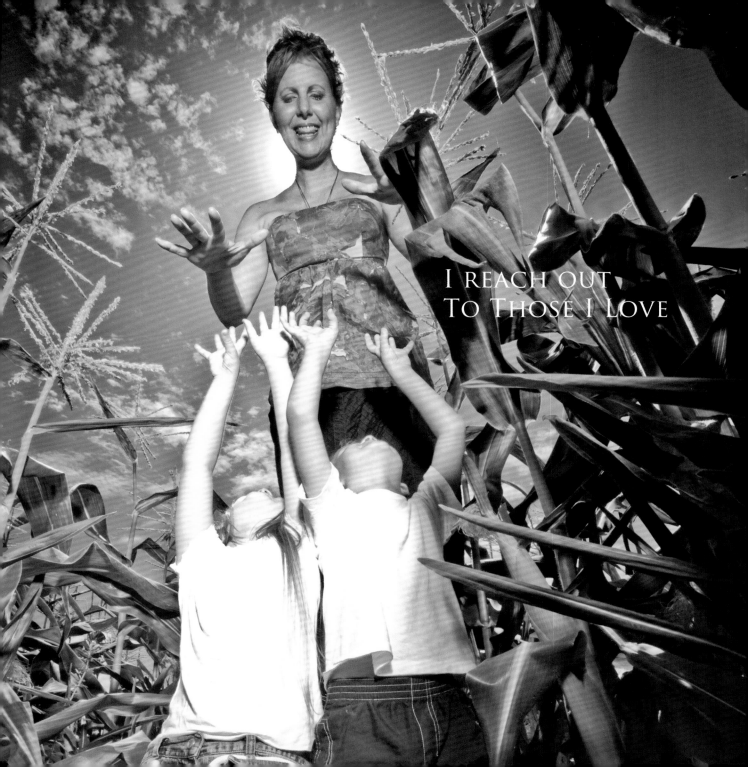

I reach out
To those I love

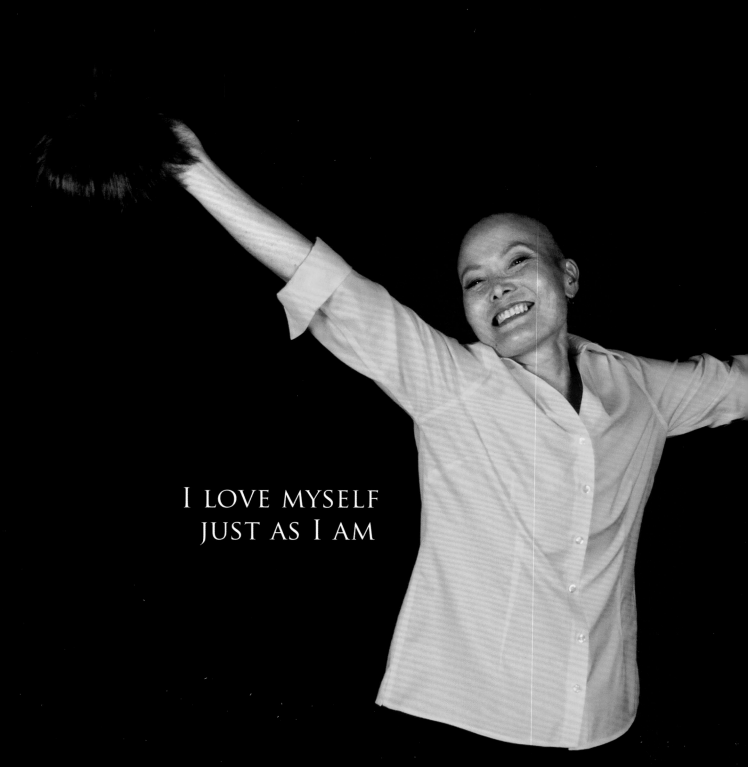

I LOVE MYSELF
JUST AS I AM

I lost my hair and gained perspective

As an oncology nurse I spent long hours at work and my priorities were to be the best, most productive I could be. I demanded the same of everyone else. I worried a lot and the fear of getting cancer was always on my mind. My fears came true. I found out I had invasive cancer of the worst kind. My entire breast was cancerous and the cancer had spread.

When I first lost all my hair, my eyebrows, and my breasts, I felt ugly. So, I bought a bunch of expensive makeup to make myself feel better. I had a wig, but it was itchy and really uncomfortable, and I hated it.

Driving home one day, I suddenly noticed how beautiful the Koʻolau mountains were. Something inside me spoke: I had been so busy trying to do everything and be my very best, I hadn't seen this great big beautiful thing I drove past every day. Cancer was God's way of getting my attention, saying, "Stop, look around, appreciate the beauty of people and the world around you." I saw how the people I had been most critical of, were the ones who loved and supported me most. I understood that while our society admires perfection, our lives are NOT perfect. I realized that what's beautiful is our hearts and souls, not the outside stuff.

So I thought, "To heck with it, I am a cancer patient and I have no hair. This is who I am, and I'm not covering it up!" I went back to work without a wig and my head uncovered. When other women in the hospital saw me, they took off their wigs too. I felt so liberated!

I've lived more in this year since my diagnosis and mastectomy than any time prior to it. I've learned to let go. Let go of trying to be perfect, of expecting others to be perfect, of judging. I stopped worrying about what other people think or do, or about what will happen in the future. Worrying didn't make me healthy, worrying didn't cure me, and worrying didn't make me or anyone else happy. So now I just don't. I feel so free and so happy. I just focus on what really matters: life and love.

~ April Goya

God keeps His promises

I broke down crying when I found out that I had breast cancer and needed surgery. I've never had so much as a broken bone, never had to stay overnight at a hospital, much less need surgery, and the whole concept overwhelmed and frightened me.

I was raised going to church, so I immediately prayed to God. Then I turned to my Bible studies lessons plan for the day. It was especially appropriate: Psalm 6:9 "The Lord hears and accepts your prayers," and James 5:14-15 " Is anyone of you sick? He should call the elders of the church to pray over him...And the prayer offered in faith will make the sick person well." These were His promises to me and answers to my prayers. I heard Him speak to me to call a friend to pick me up and take me to church to see our pastor's wife, Ruby, who was a breast cancer survivor. She organized a prayer circle for me.

Having people surrounding me and praying for me was a humbling experience. I felt so loved, so cared for and so grateful. My heart softened and I broke down sobbing. God had promised me I would be healed, but He didn't say it would be miraculous and simply disappear. I knew I had to do the work, have the surgery and go through the process, but with the support and strength and love from Ruby, all the people who prayed for me, and God, I knew I would make it through. I know God keeps His promises and if you have faith, He will never leave you.

I know it sounds funny to say this, but cancer was the best thing to ever happen to me. I have learned so much and felt love like I never had before. I know deep in my heart that if I ask for help, God will hear me and I will receive it. God keeps His promises.

~ Deb Lamb

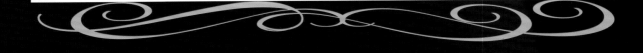

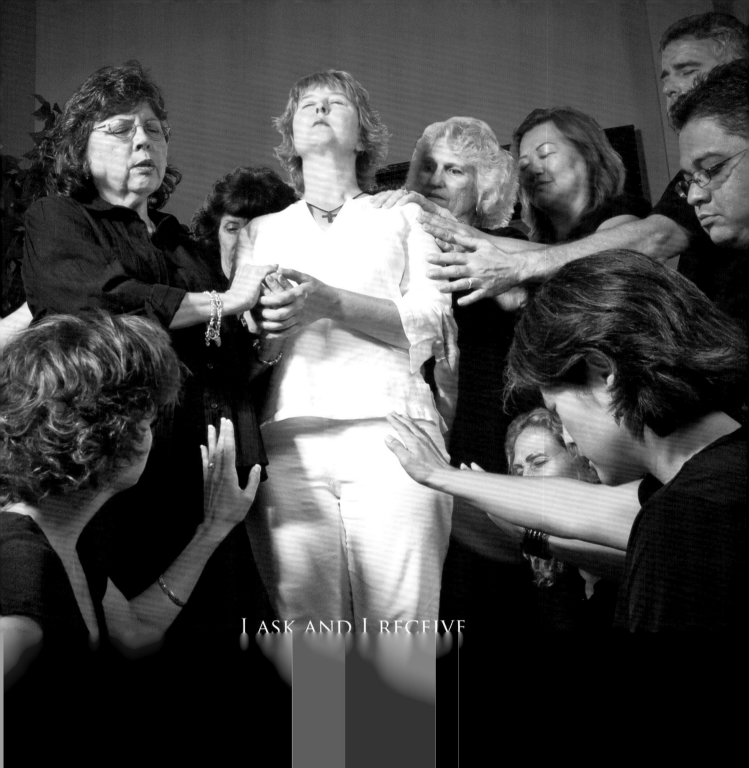

I ASK AND I RECEIVE

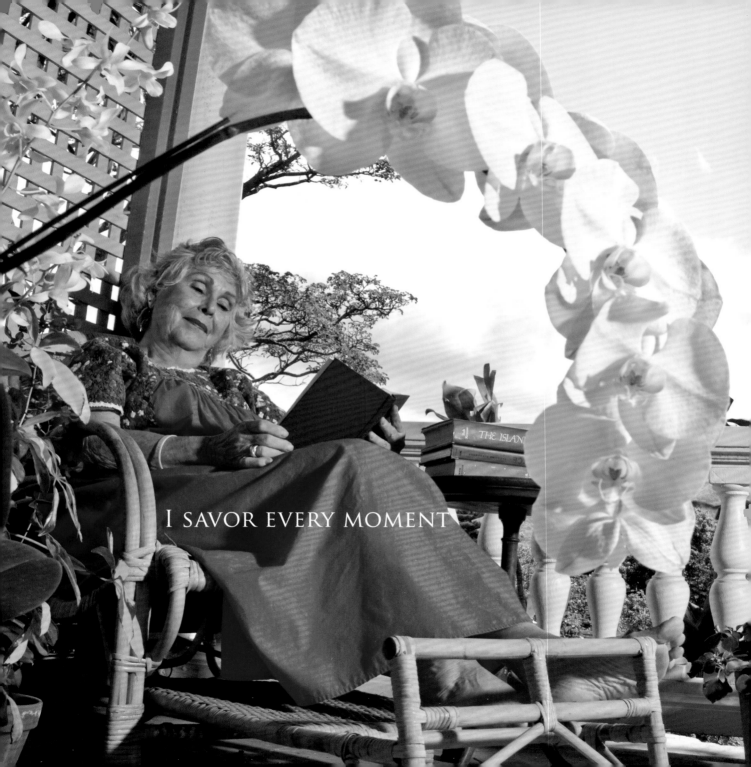

I SAVOR EVERY MOMENT

LIFE IS A STRING OF MOMENTS

At 64, I discovered a lump in my breast one day while I was soaping in the shower. I knew my body so well that I knew it wasn't good but I didn't let myself run away into the future fearing all that could go wrong. I knew what I needed to do in the immediate moment, called my doctor, then trusted in the process. I just took it one step at a time.

When I was much younger, I lived my life with a lot of fear. And being afraid didn't always lead to the best choices. So, I began to develop my spiritual self and came to see that there really is nothing to be afraid of. I learned to survive a lot of personal traumas and challenges by accepting that there are many things in life that I'm not in charge of. Over the years, I've come to accept that I don't run the show, I just take directions, hold on, and try to enjoy the ride. Moments pass and we go on.

The first couple of weeks were the scariest. I had a lumpectomy and 22 lymph nodes were removed. When I got stressed, or hit a difficult spot, I would do something to shift my focus; I'd read something inspirational like the writings of the Dalai Lama, or go to a support group meeting and would keep myself in the present moment. Instead of feeling sorry for myself, I'd find some way to give back to others. Being centered in myself, rather than being self-centered gave me a lot of strength and comfort.

This disease could easily have taken my life, but instead it gave me the opportunity to grow even more spiritually. I live my life with gratitude. Every morning I wake up grateful to see another day and I say "Thank you." In the life of the spirit, we are always at the beginning, everyday is a chance to start living again. It's true, life really is a journey and the little moments add up. At 75 years old, I'm looking forward to many more days, and many more wonderful moments.

~ LANI MURRAY

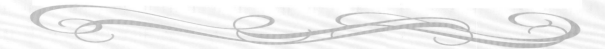

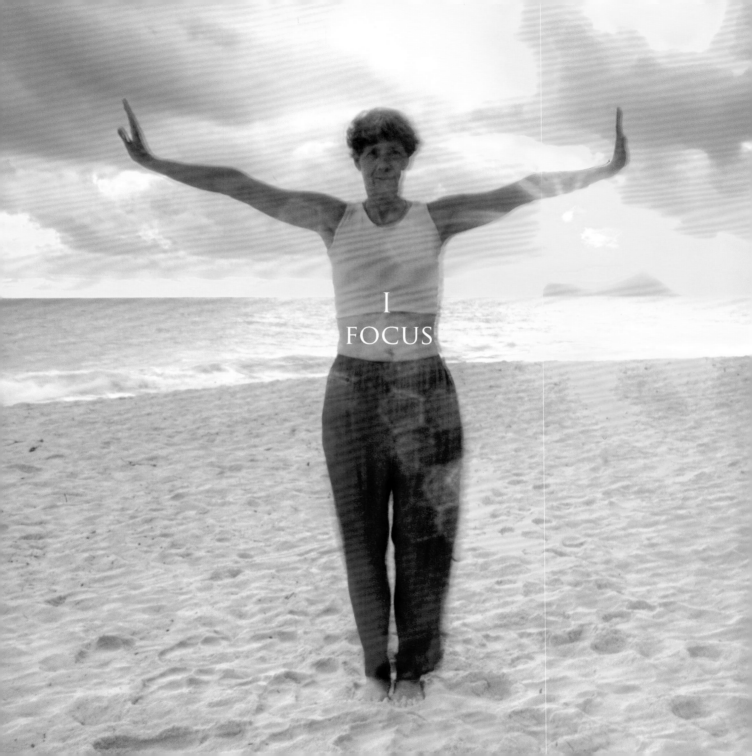

I

FOCUS

When I talk to my body, my body listens

As a former Olympic candidate, I've always been very health conscious. I was shocked when doctors told me I had Stage 3 breast cancer that had been developing for 8-10 years and it required immediate and aggressive attention.

Although I believed in the mind-body connection, I couldn't find a treatment my MIND was convinced would work. So I combined chemo with alternative approaches. I worked hard to keep a positive attitude and it paid off. I endured several radical surgery and treatments (one of them is obsolete since it's survival rate was only 1 in 100!) and I always came out better than most.

After one particularly difficult treatment, a miracle occurred: looking in the mirror at my wounded body I felt this deep love and compassion. I wiped my tears pressing a hot washcloth against my skin the way a mother would bathe an infant. Afterwards, I felt lighter and energized. The next morning, the nurses were shocked to see that my blood counts had risen from 600 to 7,700 with no sign of infection or fever. The next day my counts had doubled! I was released in two days, less than half the normal time!

I later learned from my acupuncturist that I had helped myself heal by using my own Chi. I had performed Chi-Lel™ Qigong so I began to study and practice. Wherever I sent my Chi, the pain disappeared. I began to use it during my radiation treaments and surprised the therapists when I had no burns or redness typically seen in other patients. They said to me, "Whatever you're doing, it's working! Keep going!" and I did.

I practice Chi-Lei Qigong daily and I've been cancer-free for 10 years. I haven't needed to see a doctor ever since. My body is stronger than ever and my energy is steady and full. And now I have something to give: I teach and help others heal with Chi. When we talk to our bodies, our bodies listen. This is the wisdom and power of Chi-Lel.

~ Ginny Walden

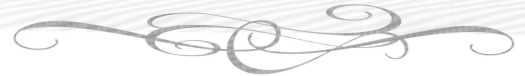

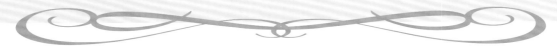

THE BEAT GOES ON ... I WILL NOT LOSE

Growing up as a small Asian kid in a military family, I learned to accept change and adapt quickly, but I always felt I had something to prove. My grandmother always said I had a hard head. I admit I never accept the idea that I can't do something, and I hate losing. I thrive on challenges. The bigger the challenge, the harder I push myself. Fighting cancer was no different.

I never did self-exams and being small, it never occurred to me that I should. At 28, I began to feel tired a lot. I started losing weight and my body just didn't feel right. When I began having sharp stabbing pains in my breast I went to the doctor and discovered I had a Stage 4 carcinoma. The medical staff was supportive, but they were clear that my chances of survival weren't good. When I heard that the odds were against me, a switch flipped in my mind. Cancer became a challenger that was out to beat me and there was no way I would let it. I made it a mission to keep my routine and gave myself the challenge of seeing how long I could go without anyone knowing about my condition.

I went through radiation and chemo and went to work even when I felt sick. I pushed through my workouts and sometimes did more just to prove that cancer wasn't winning. I expected that I'd have to tell everyone about my cancer when my hair fell out, but I found that I'm one of the few people that don't lose hair from chemo. As a result, I kept it a secret and most people never knew that I was ill. I felt like I had won in a big way.

I've been in remission for 14 years, but I know cancer is never cured and it can reappear at any time. Taiko is a powerful inspiration for me to be able to continue on. In Taiko, we embrace *kaizen*, which means change. You drum knowing that the patterns and rhythms might change unexpectedly. So you're always prepared to adapt to keep it together and keep playing. Everything in Taiko is big – the drums, the *bachi* sticks, the movements and the sound. But when you focus and put your whole being into it, even the smallest person can create mighty results.

~ CLAIRE TONG

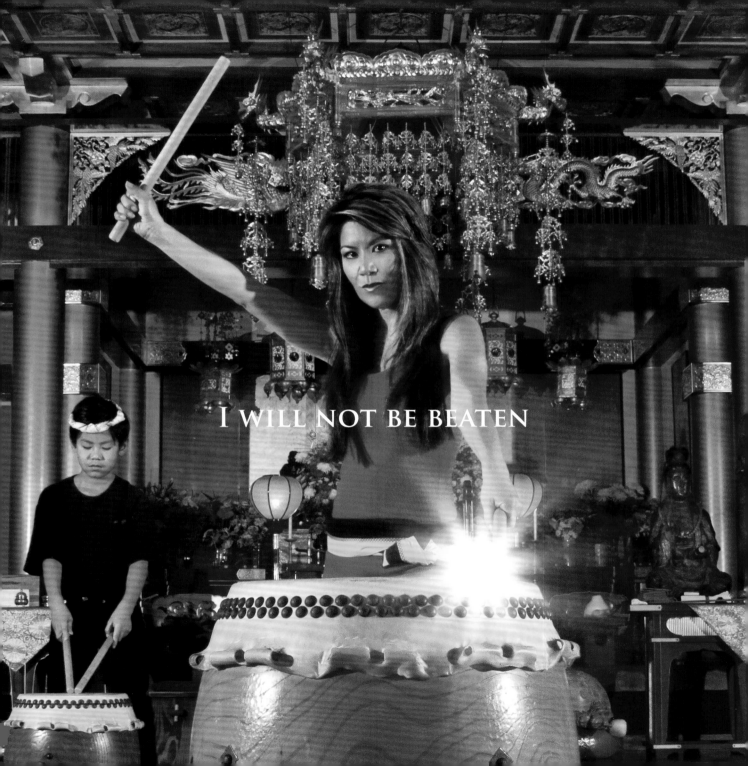

I WILL NOT BE BEATEN

I OPENED UP TO OTHERS AND FOUND MYSELF

Before I was diagnosed with breast cancer I was a total workaholic. I dedicated myself to my work, my husband, and my kids. I never took time for myself. I've always been very shy and timid and I was totally uncomfortable talking about personal issues. Cancer changed me.

When I first found out I had breast cancer I totally freaked out. I was hysterical and so convinced I was going to die, I wouldn't let the nurse go. I knew nothing about cancer and didn't realize how much help is out there. My nurse told me, "You can't just sit and dwell on this, you have to go out and do something." Then she referred me to a support group. I was totally resistant to going but I forced myself and it changed everything.

In my first group session, I found comfort and strength from absolute strangers. Woman after woman shared her very personal story. They showed me their scars, shared tips on how to wear scarves during chemo and each one encouraged me to be strong. They were so open and giving I stopped feeling embarrassed or ashamed to talk about my issues. They became my sisters and before I knew it, I really got out there. Suddenly the introvert turned into a gym-going, kick-boxing, yoga practitioner and hula student.

Of all the things I explored, hula touched me the most. My kumu taught me that the key to hula is to feel the story from the inside so it can find expression on the outside. I learned to move with spirit and dance with emotion.

I'm still a bit shy, but now I'm able to express myself in ways I never could before. I perform with my hula sisters in Waikiki and I even wear sparkles to work sometimes. The world is brighter now that I've learned the power of my spirit to overcome. I'm over the hump. I'm a survivor.

~ DALE TANIMOTO

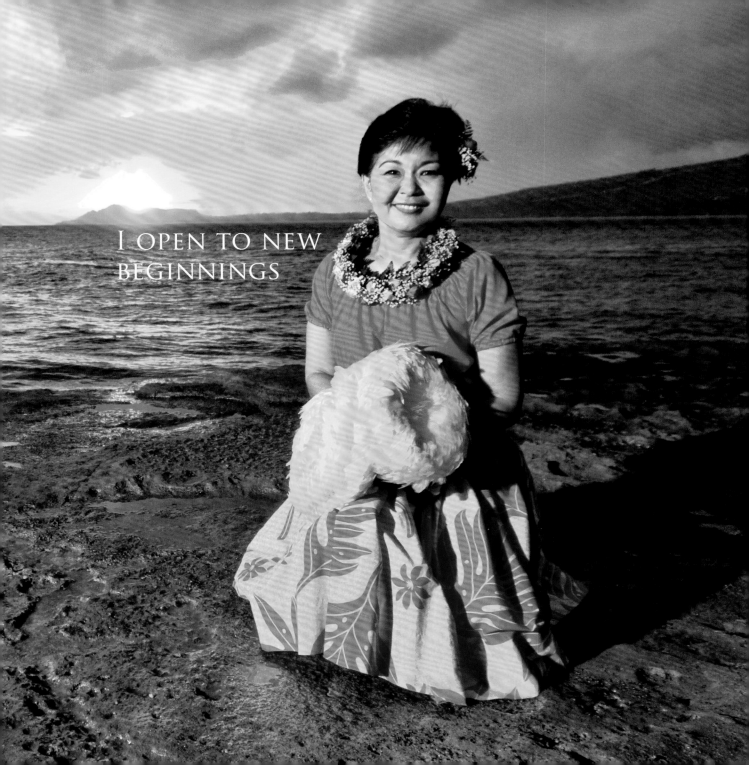

I OPEN TO NEW
BEGINNINGS

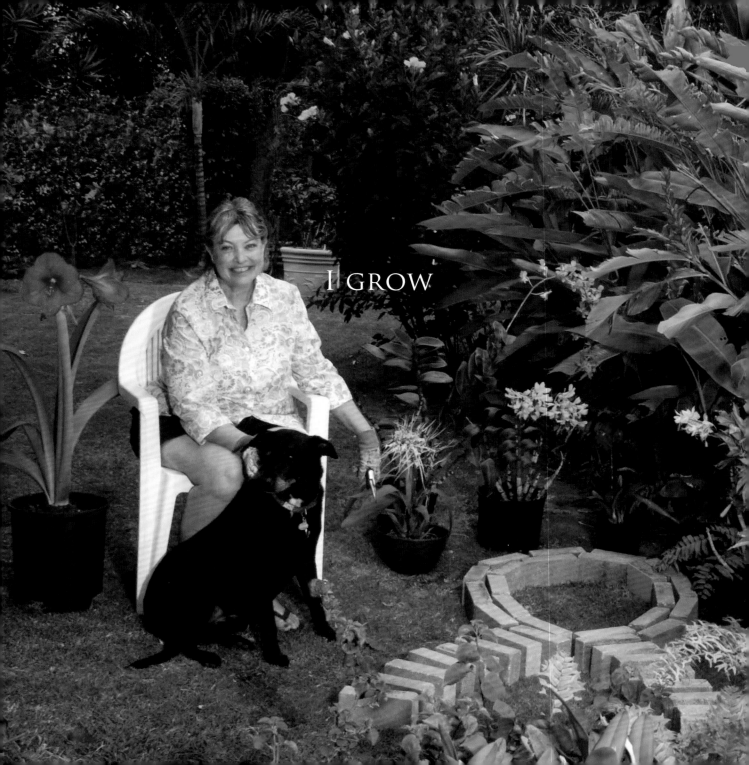

I GROW

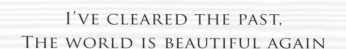

I'VE CLEARED THE PAST,
THE WORLD IS BEAUTIFUL AGAIN

I come from a large family. Both of my parents each had eight siblings and I have fifty-six first cousins. What's crazier is that sixteen members of my family have had breast cancer and only four have survived. Today the survival rates have gone up to about eighty-five percent, because we have the technology and awareness to identify and treat it.

I tested positive for the BRCA II gene so I knew cancer was in my future. It wasn't a question of "if" I would get cancer but "when." Still, when I heard my tumor was malignant, I had to grip my doctor's desk to keep from falling out of my chair.

When my treatments began, we were remodeling our home interior but I felt best working outside. Before we had moved in, part of our property had been used as a dump. There were car parts, furniture, oil drums, you name it. It was a horrible mess but I loved clearing out the junk and visualizing how I was going to make a beautiful garden.
I felt so good seeing how I could transform something and bring beauty into the world.

I believe in the power of our minds. Illness results when our minds and spirits are out of alignment. I knew that if I had a wellness attitude I could play an active role in my own healing. I dug deep within myself then wept as I realized how I had allowed fifty years to pile on me. I had lost that wonderful life-loving spirit I was as a child. Instead, I carried years of repressed anger and resentments. I needed to drop them. So I wrote a healing affirmation for myself and began planting seeds inside myself just as I did in my garden outside. And as I cleared out my yard, I also imagined my body being cleared of cancer.

The first time someone said to me, "Someday, you'll see your cancer is a gift," I wanted to punch him out. But now I see he was right. I've cleared out all my internal junk, got rid of toxic people and unhealthy situations. I know when to say "no" and tend to myself. I'm cancer-free and joyful again. I love my life. And my garden is growing beautifully.

~ JULIE PURCELL

I lost my baggage and found my flow

Over twenty years ago breast cancer was considered a "woman thing" and not talked about openly. It was awkward when I told my family and coworkers about my cancer and little was said in response. The fear and isolation was overwhelming. I prayed for help and was amazed when complete strangers, friends of friends, offered to help me. I learned that the universe will support you. Help may not come from where you expect, but it comes if you ask and are open to receiving it.

My father was a farmer and he taught me that to really cure a disease, whether it was in a plant, animal or human, I had to look deeply and find the cause and conditions that create and support the disease. So after my surgery, I took six months off from work to really examine my life and my internal emotional systems. I opened to many different healing practices and found they had similar principles: love yourself and others, and forgive yourself and others for who they are and who they are not. I realized that it was time to let go of my emotional baggage and the toxic thoughts I carried from my past.

Snorkeling trained me to let go. I loved floating and being so light and buoyant. Feeling the tingle of currents on my skin and seeing all the vivid colors of corals and fish gave me a wonderful sense of peace. I felt so free. But, if I was preoccupied and caught up in my mind, I'd miss a gorgeous fish, or get swept out to sea or thrown into rocks by waves or currents. Whenever my thoughts drifted to unreasonable expectations, worries, frustrations, resentments or anger, I would breathe, focus and let them go. When I came back to shore they would be gone, washed away. Snorkeling was a gift.

Cancer was my turning point and it transformed me. Now I take better care of myself and I pay close attention to my thoughts and emotions. I see how we all have choices and thoughts create reality, so staying positive is a great opportunity. Why dwell on negative issues and load yourself with baggage when you can glide through life and enjoy the views? Life is wonderful when you let go and flow.

~ Jane Yamashiro

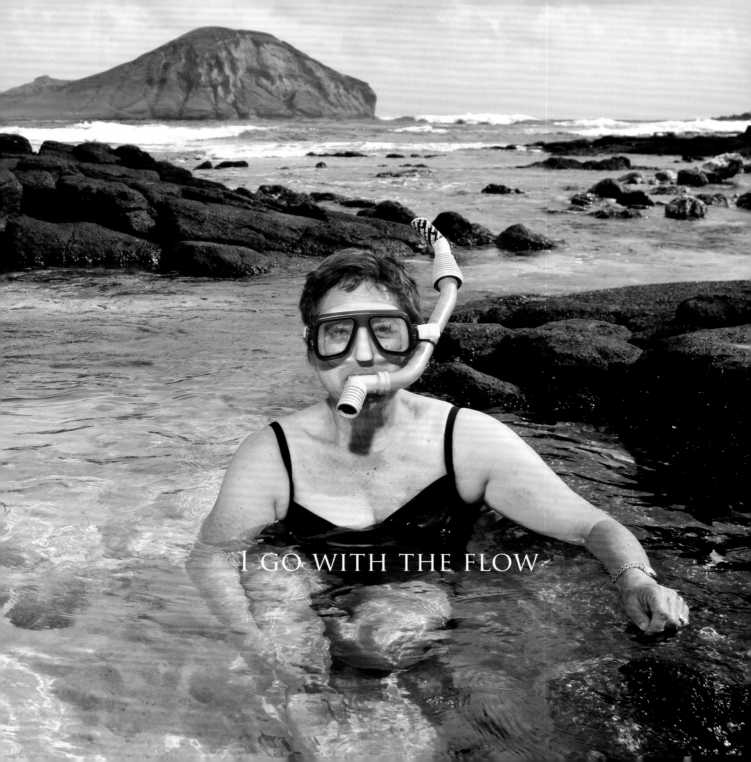

I GO WITH THE FLOW

Bling bling, it's all good

My mother had breast cancer 30 years ago and it never crossed my mind that I might get it too. When she went through it, she held it together and always looked immaculate. She survived and we never dwelled on it. When I was diagonosed, I followed her lead.

As the oldest child, I'm used to being the one in charge, the one who takes care of things and makes others laugh when times get tough. Being around positive people in positive environments keeps me strong, so I always try to surround myself with happy energy.

Going to the oncologist was terrible. The doctor and staff were great, but sitting in the dull colored waiting rooms with so many sick patients depressed me. I hated it. So I took charge. The first thing I did was jump online and learn everything I could about breast cancer. Then I started managing my doctors and schedules like I managed my job. I played with appointment times until I figured out when I'd spend the least amount of time in their offices. Then I persuaded my doctors to coordinate my tests so I could have them done in one office appointment and they would share the results. I did everything I could to stay out of their drab offices and in my "happy place."

I needed to surround myself with light and life but as a banker my workday clothes were always conservative, low key, and totally unlike me. When I was going through raditation I decided to wear bright colors to my docotor appointments to keep me feeling bright and cheery. My clothing became the antidote to the dreary and depressing waiting rooms. I started with a wildly colorful blouse and to my surprise, everyone loved it. Within weeks, I was wearing bright colors, bling sparkles and sequins everyday. My crazy "unbanker-like" outfits became entertainment for my co-workers and great fun for me. I loved it!

Cancer was a reminder of how lucky I am to have such positive and supportive people in my family and in my life. My cancer is gone now and except for my surgery scars, nothing's really changed except my wardrobe. I'll keep buying sparkly outfits. I love being the bling banker and letting my fun, bright, shiny self show!

~ Anna Marie Springer

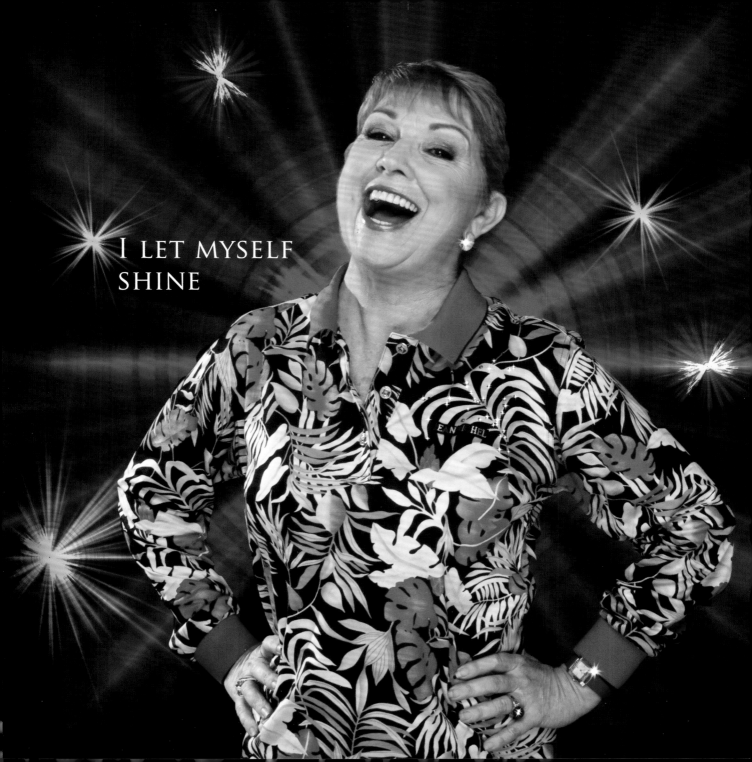

I LET MYSELF
SHINE

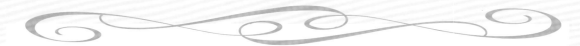

Help is there when you need it

I've been very blessed in so many ways. Although I've never taken anything for granted, I never thought breast cancer would happen to me. I had always kept in shape and took good care of myself. Whenever I had my hair done with Henry, I'd see breast cancer patients coming in to get their head shaved and have a wig styled for them. I never imagined I'd become one of them.

I had a history of fibrocysctic breasts which made them lumpy and difficult for me to do self-exams. So as a precaution, I made appointments with a breast specialist every three months. One day, I found a lump that was different from the others. After a whirlwind of ultrasounds, CAT scans, x-rays and biopsies we found a carcinoma in my left breast and on my right kidney.

The whole chemo experience is very stressful but you find ways to get through it. It's surprising how much help is out there. People I didn't know would offer me their prayers and support. The doctors and hospital staff were exceptionally kind and caring, and helped me make the best decisions. My family and friends sprung into action to support me, and my daughter temporarily left her job in New York City to be with me.

Losing my hair was very traumatic. I went straight to Henry who chose a wig for me and styled it beautifully. He made me look and feel human again, and it made a big difference for me emotionally. "Look good to feel good" is his motto, and I agree.

I'm grateful I was diligent in getting examined, and good things have come from my experience. My daughter now produces major fund raising events supporting breast cancer patients. And my husband and I continue to grow closer in our 42 years of marriage. If I've learned anything, it's that every woman needs to have regular breast exams. Whether she does them herself or has help, she needs to do it as often as possible. It makes a difference.

~ Madeline Scherman

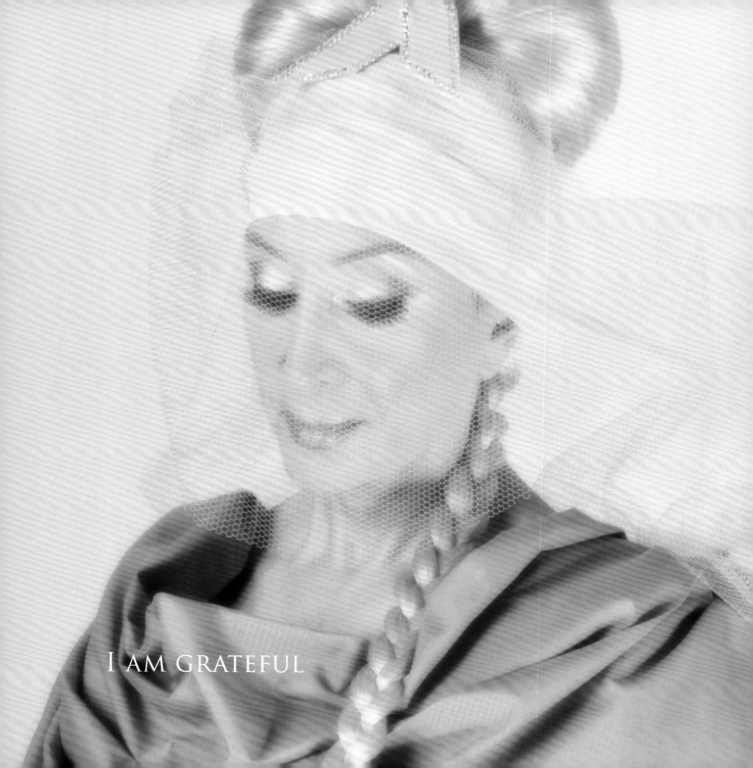

I AM GRATEFUL

Embraced by Angels

My mother was my comforter and I could always rely on her. Before she passed away, she told me, "Don't cry too much. I can do more for you from the other side than I can on this side." At the time, I didn't understand what she meant.

When I found a lump it my breast I panicked. I was deathly afraid of the "C" word. My family tried to reassure me and get me to a doctor, but I absolutely refused. So they had to trick me. One night my sisters invited me for a ride to pick up my niece and before I knew it, they were walking me into a hospital emergency room.

I was diagnosed with Stage 3 cancer and I totally fell apart. All I wanted was my mother, so my husband drove me to her grave. When I knelt down and prayed for her help, something caressed me. I felt as if I were being embraced in a warm hug. I could feel my mother's presence and that's when I understood what she meant all those years before. I knew my mother was with me as my angel and I would be okay.

I was overwhelmed with love and support. My coworkers created a fund to help pay for my treatment and relieved much of my financial stress. My sisters were amazing. After a round of chemo, my sister offered to help me wash my hair. As she ran her fingers over my head every strand of hair fell out. I had no idea it was happening until she began weeping and hugged me tightly. She said, "I love you and I want you to know you are beautiful no matter what. If you want, I'll shave my head right now and be bald with you." We cried together and I felt completely loved.

Throughout my healing, I prayed to God and my angels when I needed comfort. Sometimes I'd go outside to admire God's creation, the mountains, the ocean and the moon, and reconnect to the sensation of being held by angels. Cancer helped me find my spirit and my strength. My husband tells me I'm a strong woman. I say, "Of course I am, I have God, my family, and my mother at my side!"

~ Lehua King

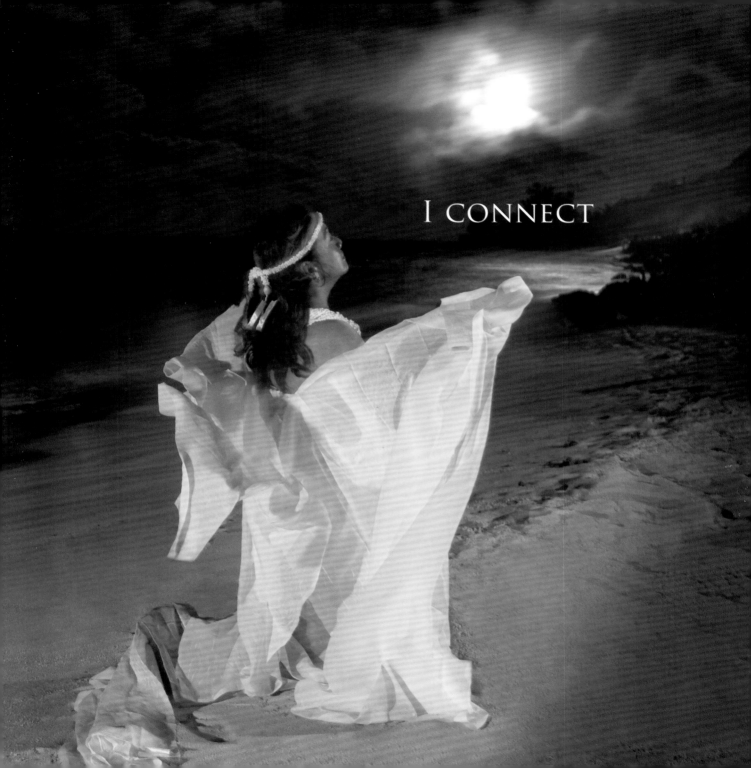

I CONNECT

Peace in passion

I never thought cancer would ever happen to me. The idea of death and dying was something that I was so afraid of I couldn't even think about it. I grew up in the Catholic church and had always attended mass regularly but the idea of an afterlife had seemed so abstract and far off. When I was diagnosed with Stage 1 breast cancer I was suddenly faced with the reality of my own mortality.

During my chemo treatments I felt as if I were dying, and in some respects I was. Chemotherapy kills the bad cancer cells, but it also takes down good cells too. I felt like I was clutching onto my life by a thread, I couldn't eat but I know I needed to in order to survive and heal.

One Sunday at church as I was accepting the Eucharist, I looked at the wine and I thought of the chemo cocktail I had just consumed to kill my cancer cells. Now I was consuming wine and bread, Jesus' blood and body, to protect my good cells and help me heal. Jesus had survived and his blood was now flowing through me...in that moment my faith and the story of Jesus' passion became real for me. I felt the grace of God's peace and knew I would be safe.

Cancer gave me a deeper appreciation of life and my faith. Through my treatments and healing, I came to understand the power of Jesus in a very personal way. I'm a survivor. I'm not afraid anymore.

~ Caroline Huff

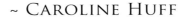

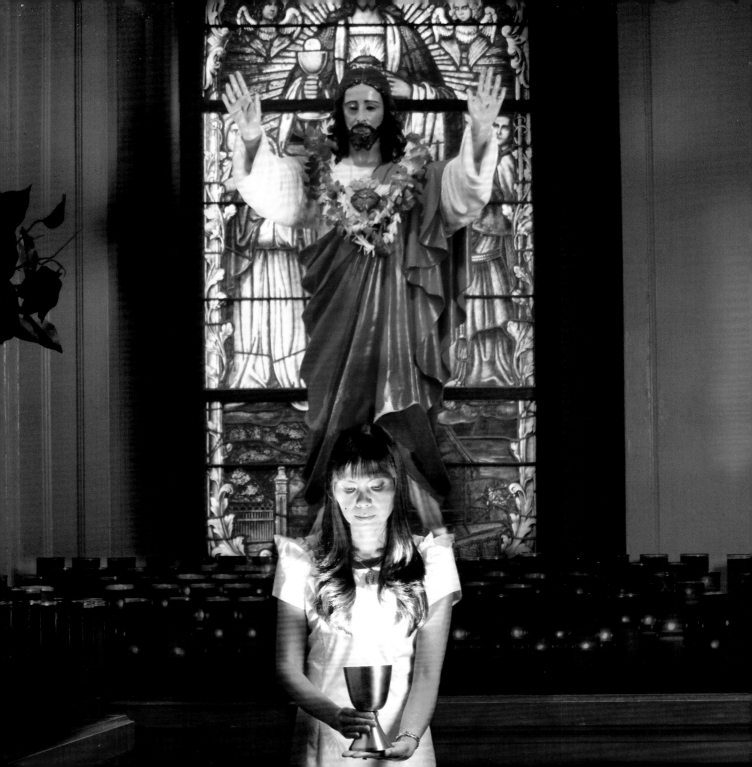

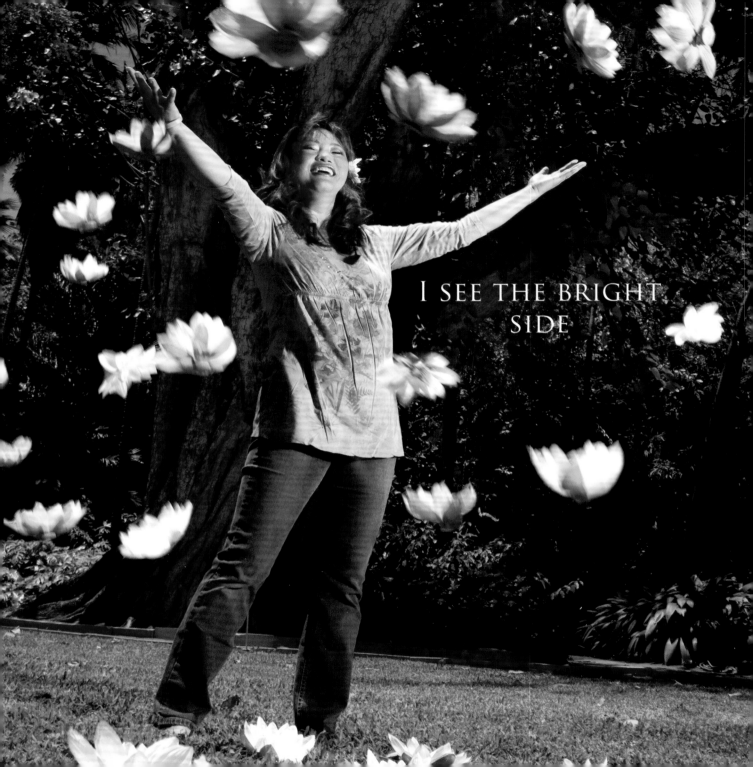

I SEE THE BRIGHT
SIDE

Out of muck, flowers bloom

Initially, I refused to have a mammogram. I had no family history of breast cancer nor any lumps in my breasts. I was only thirty-eight and I wanted to wait until I was forty, when it's a standard procedure. But I accepted my doctor's suggestion and had one.

When they found cancer I was ecstatic! It was very small, between Stage 0 and Stage 1, and was much easier to treat than if I had waited the two years to find it. I felt so incredibly lucky that we found it early, I was giddy. I was at a time in my life where I was "cleaning house" and starting fresh. I had just gotten a divorce, accepted a new job, and was leaving a difficult time behind me. Having my "tiny" cancer removed just seemed like one more step to a happier, healthier life and I was glad to take it.

I checked in for my surgery one morning and was out by that afternoon. Radiation treatments followed. I had a few minor complications and discomforts, but they passed quickly and I continued to revel in the fact that it could have been much worse. Over the course of my treatments I got to know my doctor and her staff really well and we always had something to laugh about. I felt like I was winning in life and nothing could dampen my spirits.

As a Buddhist I understand that life isn't always easy. I also believe that we can transform a negative experience into a positive one. Throughout my treatments and to this day I chant "Nam-myoho-renge-kyo" daily. "Renge" literally means "lotus flower," and it reminds us that like the lotus flower, we can rise above the swamp in our lives and blossom. No matter how difficult or challenging our lives may be, we can overcome the hardship and something beautiful can emerge from it.

Through my experience, I've been able to help others. And I'm a testament to the value of mammograms and early detection. I see my cancer as a blessing. It marks a time in my life when I was reminded of how beautiful life can be. I'm so happy to be alive!

~ Sharon Ogata

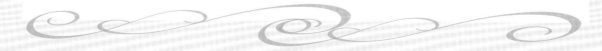

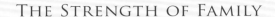

THE STRENGTH OF FAMILY

I know it sounds strange, but when I found out I had cancer, I wasn't devastated. I was always really good about getting regular check ups and I figured we found it early enough. We've suffered so many shocking passings in my family, from my parents, my brothers Gerald, Fred and Eddie, to my young nephews Eddie-Boy and Clyde Jr. that I think I'm numb to the idea of dying.

Still, I prayed to my parents, "Can you help me out?" and somehow inside, I just knew I would be okay. I could feel the strength of my mother and father's love and I felt them watching over me. And with them, comes the rest of my ohana. Everybody knows how loving, caring and brave Eddie was. If you look closely, you'll see that everything he was, everything he did, came from our parents. We were taught to take care of everybody, especially each other.

During my treatment, my brothers moved back into the house to be with me. I kept expecting to be really sick, but I never really felt as bad as I thought I would. I was weak and in pain after my surgery but I was never bored, never went hungry, and was never alone. My brothers cooked for me every night and made sure I was comfortable. If I got stir crazy, one of my brothers would take me for a drive, or the family would make a *lū'au* and we'd sing and have a big party. One day my baby brother Clyde walked in the house with his head totally shaved and made me laugh. He said, "I like my head match yours! As long as you look like dat, I goin look like dis!" He kept it shaved until my hair grew back. I was shocked at first but not really surprised, that's just how we are.

We never had a lot of money, but we are rich in family and love. We did everything together. We are so tight, when one is hurt, all of us feel it. Together we were bigger than my cancer, and the pain was little compared to all the love I have. Now I help others get through their cancer and keep doing what comes naturally in my family: just live aloha and love everybody.

~ MYRA AIKAU

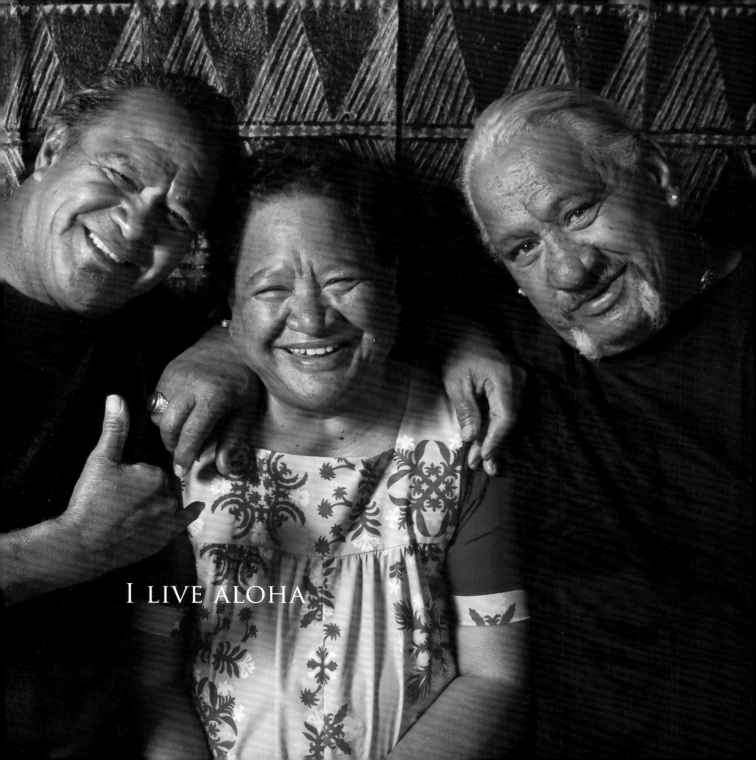

I live aloha

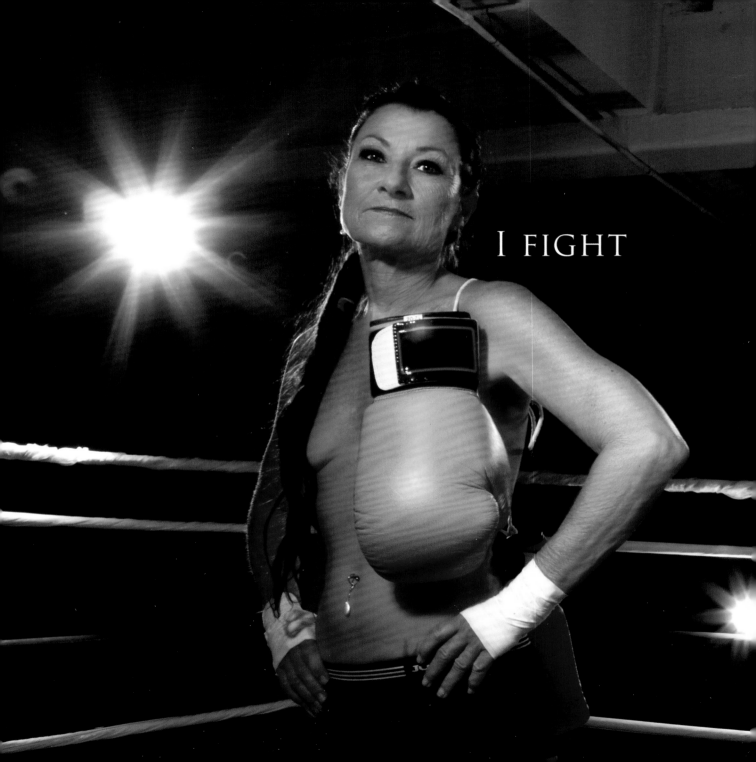

I FIGHT

Take a licking, keep on ticking

My story is unusual but it's proof that you can survive anything. My long journey with cancer began 30 years ago. I was in the military assigned to a Nuclear Biological Chemical Warfare Team. As a radiation technician, I was exposed to high levels of toxic chemicals and radiation. Within a year of leaving the service, I was diagnosed with breast cancer.

I had surgery and did chemo and was "clear" of cancer, but a year later, another form of cancer arose. I beat it. Then a few years later, another cancer appeared and I beat that. This just went on and on, but I'm still here. I took the lickings and kept on ticking!

Beating cancer isn't always pretty. Aside from the physical aspects, there are difficulties on many levels. Back then, we knew so little about cancer, hearing you had it was like getting a death sentence. No one would really talk about it. Some of the people closest to me were so convinced that I was dying they disappeared from my life, because they didn't want to watch it happen and didn't know what to do. And, the treatments can drain you financially.

At first I cried, "Why me?" Then I thought, "Why not me? What makes me think I'm so special that this could happen to someone else and not to me?" I stopped feeling sorry for myself. I asked, "What is the gift in all this?" I realized that I was strong and I could handle it, and I could help others who might not be as strong. I decided that I am a SURVIVOR and my life purpose is bigger than whatever moment of suffering I have to face.

I've been told twice that I only had 90 days to live. All it did was make me mad. No one has the right to tell you when your time is up, and I knew it wasn't my time. I survived and proved them wrong. I never compromise in my belief that I'm NOT going to die.

Over the past three decades, I've conquered brain tumors, skin cancer, uterine cancer and repeated rounds of breast cancer. I survived them all. If it happens again, I'll kick that one too. I don't see problems, I just see challenges. I never say "dying," I just keep fighting. I have a purpose in this world and my work is not done.

~ Kate Wagner

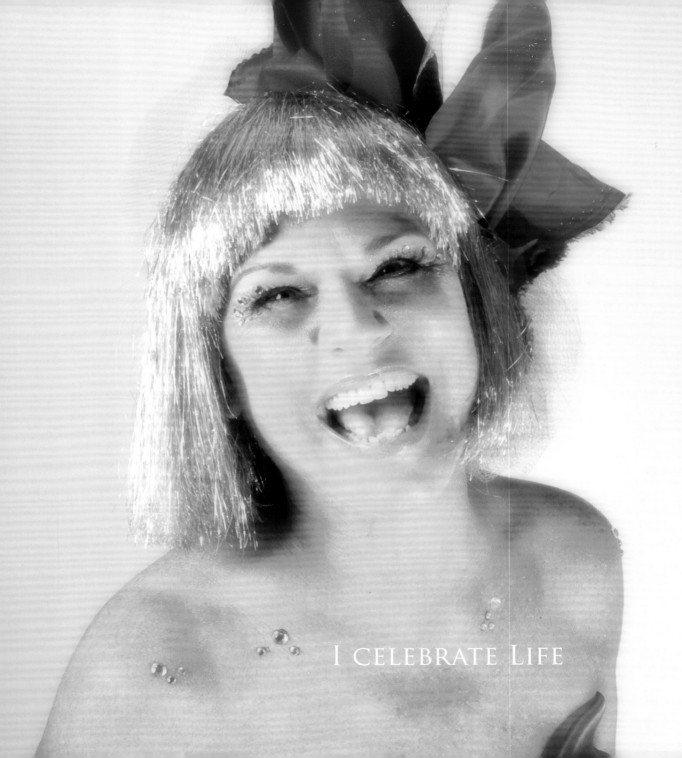

I celebrate Life

NEVER STOP LAUGHING

I was transformed the day I was diagnosed with breast cancer. I walked into the doctor's office a "normal person" and walked out an official member of what I call the "Big Pink Ribbon Society." I was given a giant pink canvas bag full of breast cancer information and materials. I felt like I was back in school with a ton of homework! I had a lot of options to explore and decisions to make. I had a clue about what I was in for, but I wasn't going to let it beat me down. We caught it early and that was something to celebrate.

Losing my hair was very traumatic but I still found things to laugh about. A lot of women take control, shave their heads and get a wig right off the bat. I figured I'd let it fall out on it's own and keep what I could. At one point I looked like a little old man with little white springs instead of a comb-over. The flip side was I never worried about getting a crappy hair cut and I still don't. Being bald is funny when you don't think about all the heavy stuff.

Whenever I was home I'd take my wig off and toss it anywhere. From a distance it looked like a big fuzzy animal so we started referring to it as my pet, "Sparky." Sparky was great at helping me go out without feeling self-conscious, but he wasn't always so well behaved. My husband and I laugh about the times I hadn't paid attention when Sparky slipped or shifted, and I'd be circulating at a party or event with what looked like a really bad cock-eyed haircut.

Don't get me wrong, the whole process of battling breast cancer is very traumatic, tiring and stressful. It will slow you down, but don't ever let it stop you, don't let it beat you. My husband and I learned the cycles during my treatments and we made sure to make my "I feel okay" times a celebration. We'd plan weekend getaways and special trips, and I started the whole thing with a special shopping trip to the mainland with my best friends. Life is good. Keep laughing, keep your spirits up and never, ever, ever give up.

~ NOMA McLELLAN

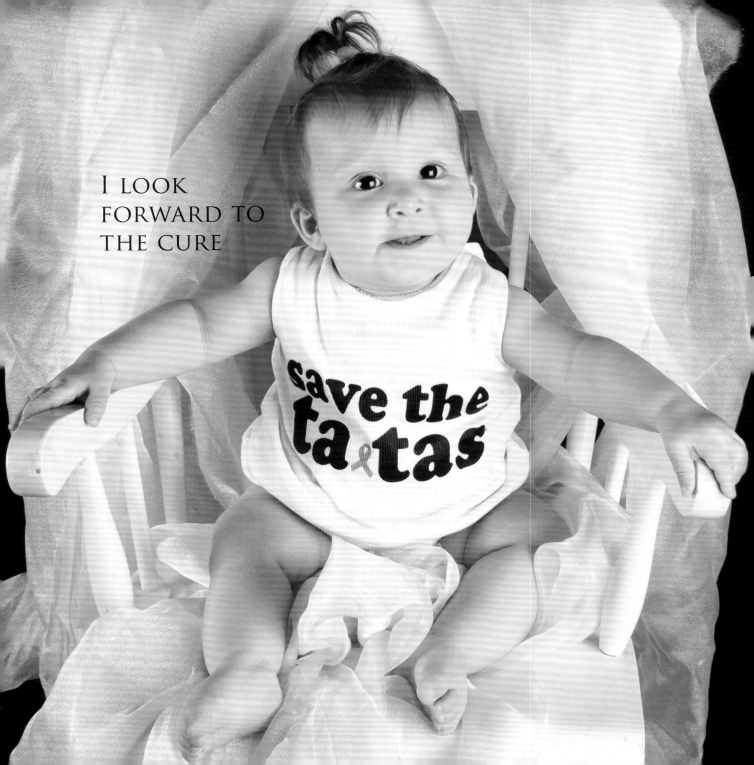

I LOOK
FORWARD TO
THE CURE

save the
ta tas

THRIVE IN THE POWER, PASSION,
AND BEAUTY OF YOUR SPIRIT ~
LIVE STRONG

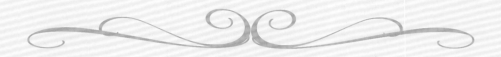

THE SURVIVOR SPIRIT
PINK PAGES

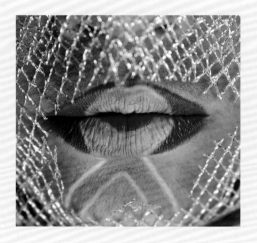

The survivors featured in this book found additional support and
information through referrals and independent research.
Following are some of their resources.

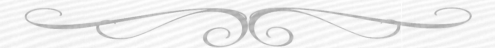

National Resources

Air Charity Network
aircharitynetwork.org
Air travel assistance for cancer patients.

American Cancer Society (ACS)
www.cancer.org
1-800-227-2345
808-595-7500 (Hawai'i Chapter)
Nationwide community-based voluntary health organization dedicated to preventing cancer, saving lives, and diminishing suffering from cancer, through research, education, advocacy, and service.

ACS Reach to Recovery program
www.cancer.org
1-800-227-2345
Breast cancer survivors mentor and assist breast cancer patients in thier recovery. Survivors volunteer to visit women in the hospital after surgery or at home once they have completed the Reach to Recovery volunteer training. This must be done with approval from both the volunteers' doctor and the patients' doctor.

Association of Community Cancer Centers
www.accc-cancer.org
See the publication "Cancer Treatments Your Insurance Should Cover."

Association of Online Cancer Reources (ACOR)
www.acor.org
1-800-227-2345
Internet-based public charity dedicated to being a reliable source of knowledge, support and community to empower those suffering from cancer. Provides uninterrupted open access to a online peer support groups (Health eCommunities). Host to a number of exceptional patient-centered websites, mailing lists and information on clinical trials.

American Society of Clinical Oncology (ASCO)
www.asco.org
The world's leading professional organization representing physicians who treat people with cancer.

Breastcancer.org
www.breastcancer.org
Dedicated to providing the most reliable, complete, and up-to-date information about breast cancer. Order free printed booklets including information about your pathology report, treatment options, and overcoming your fears.

Cancercare.org
www.cancercare.org
1- 800-813-HOPE (1-800-813-4673)
Provides free, professional support services to anyone affected by cancer: people with cancer, caregivers, children, loved ones, and the bereaved. Programs including counseling, education, financial assistance and practical help provided by trained oncology social workers completely free of charge. for diagnostic work-up, as well as information on drug assistance programs and information on transportation assistance.

Corporate Angel Network
www.corpangelnetwork.org
Air travel assistance for cancer patients

Health Care Choices
www.healthcarechoices.org
Search for information on a variety of breast cancer care issues, including patient volume data and insurance coverage.

HER2 Support Group
www.her2support.org
This unique support group provides links to news and current research for patients, caregivers, mothers, daughters, sons and husbands of breast cancer survivors who are HER2 positive.

In Your Corner
www.inyourcorner.com
Knowledge, guidance and support to help you cope.

Lance Armstrong Foundation - LiveStrong
www.laf.org
(512) 236-8820
Provides practical information, tools and support needed by people with cancer to live life on their own terms and help you face the challenges and changes that come with cancer.

Lifeline Pilots

www.airlifelinemidwest.org

Air travel assistance for cancer patients.

Living Beyond Breast Cancer

www.lbbc.org

484-708-1550

610-645-4567

Information on breast cancer treatment, testing, side effects, updates on clinical trials and the latest news on surgeries, medicines, targeted therapies and a variety of medical and quality-of-life issues.

Look Good ... Feel Better

1-800-227-2345

www.lookgoodfeelbetter.org

Volunteers provide information to women undergoing cancer treatment to help them look and feel better and be comfortable with the changes in their appearances. This program is offered by licensed cosmetologists and health care professionals.

Mercy Medical Airlift

www.mercymedical.org

Air travel assistance for cancer patients.

National Breast Cancer Foundation

www.nationalbreastcancer.org

Breast Cancer Basics including screening, prevention and treatment. Living with breast cancer and current topics in breast cancer.

National Cancer Institute

www.cancer.gov

Conducts and supports research, training, health information dissemination, and other programs with respect to the cause, diagnosis, prevention, and treatment of cancer, rehabilitation from cancer, and the continuing care of cancer patients and the families, of cancer patients. Information on risk assessment, genetic testing, participating in clinical trials.

National Coaltion for Cancer Survivorship

www.canceradvocacy.org

888-650-9127 (toll-free)

The oldest survivor-led cancer advocacy organization in the country, championing quality cancer care and empowering survivors. Provides access to credible and accurate patient information such as NCCS's award-winning Cancer Survival Toolbox® to help patients demand and receive quality care. Organizers of Cancer Advocacy Now!™, a legislative advocacy network for systemic changes in how the nation researches, regulates, finances, and delivers quality cancer care. Find help with financing issues and medical assistance. Access publications including, "Working It Out: Your Employment Rights as a Cancer Survivor," "What Cancer Survivors Need to Know About Health Insurance," and "A Cancer Survivor's Almanac: Charting Your Journey".

National Family Caregivers Association

1-800-896-3650 (Toll-Free)

www.nfcacares.org

Access the latest resources, connect with others, and find support with NFCA's Family Caregiver Community. Free information resources, and Pen Pal program which connects you directly with others who are caring for loved ones.

National Patient Air Travel HELPLINE

www.patienttravel.org

Air travel assistance for cancer patients.

National Womens Health Information Center

1-800- 994-9662 (Toll-Free)

The Federal Government Source for Women's Health Information. U. S. Department of Health and Human Services Office on Women's Health.

Network of Strength (formerly Y-Me)

www.networkofstrength.org

312-986-8338

Trusted resource for 30 years and has helped thousands find the information they need to make educated decisions. They explain in plain language the information you're likely to encounter.

Nueva Vida, Inc.

www.nueva-vida.org

202-223-9100

Information and support for Latinas whose lives are affected by cancer. Nueva Vida advocates for and facilitates the timely access to state of the art cancer care, including screening, diagnosis, treatment and care for all Latinas.

Partnership for Prescription Assistance

www.pparx.org

Drug assistance program information.

Patient Advocate Foundation

www.patientadvocate.org

Offers legal and advocacy help when disputing insurance claim denials, as well as financial assistance information.

Pauline Books & Media

www.pauline.org

1-866-521-2731 (Toll-Free)

People Living with Cancer

www.plwc.org

Patient information website of the American Society of Clinical Oncology (ASCO) is designed to help patients and families make informed health-care decisions.

Pharmaceutical Research and Manufacturers of America

www.phrma.org

Directory of pharmaceutical manufacturers' assistance programs.

Planet Cancer

www.planetcancer.org

An international network of young adult cancer patients.

Sisters Network, Inc.

www.sistersnetworkinc.org

1-866-781-1808

Information and support for African Americans affected by cancer. Sisters Network, Inc. is committed to increasing local and national attention to the devastating impact that breast cancer has in the African American community.

The Susan Komen for The Cure Foundation

www.komen.org

1-800-IM-AWARE (1-800-462-9273)

World's largest grassroots network of breast cancer survivors and activists fighting to save lives, empower people, ensure quality care for all and energize science to find the cures. Largest source of nonprofit funds dedicated to the fight against breast cancer in the world. Site includes extensive resources to answer any question regarding breast cancer and direct you to financial help, support groups and hotlines, as well as information on breast cancer prevention, risk factors and environmental links to breast cancer.

Toppers

1-800-227-2345

Work with a trained volunteer to select a wig, along with scarves and/or hats at no charge to the patient. Must be registered with the local American Cancer Society Unit office. Call to locate the ACS office nearest you for an appointment.

Young Survival Coalition

www.youngsurvival.org

1-646-257-3000

Premier international, nonprofit network with focus on awareness and education of breast cancer issues in women under 40. YSC seeks to educate the medical, research, breast cancer and legislative communities and to persuade them to address breast cancer in women 40 and under. Serves as a point of contact for young women living with breast cancer.

Your Shoes - 24/7 Breast Cancer Support Center

www.networkofstrength.org/programs/yourshoes.php

1-800-221-2141 (English)*

*Interpreters available in 150 languages

24-hours a day, talk with trained peer counselors who are survivors, patients and/or supporters who have had experience with breast cancer. Anonymous resource for breast cancer and breast health information. Support is provided to anyone touched by or concerned about this disease.

Alternative & Complementary

American Association of Naturopathic Physicians
www.naturopathic.org
Naturopathic physicians are trained in the art and science of natural healthcare at accredited medical colleges. Integrative partnerships between conventional medical doctors and licensed NDs are becoming more available. Find a licensed ND by zip code.

American Massage Therapy Association
http://www.amtamassage.org
Find an accredited AMTA licensed massage therapist. Search by state, name and/or modality.

Blue Sky Healing Arts (CHI-LEL Medical Qigong)
www.blueskyhealingarts.com
Featured survivor Ginny Walden shares her knowledge and tactics for survival and the power of CHI-LEI™ MEDICAL QIGONG to create healing. Ms. Walden trained in Beijing, China under seven top CHI-LEI™ Masters to become one of five CHI-LEI™ Senior Teachers in the world. Ginny has taught the art of self-healing to thousands of people in Hawaii and world-wide.

CancerConsultants.com
www.cancerconsultants.com
Free and confidential clinical trials matching and referral services. Daily Cancer News is the core of Cancer Consultants' educational content platform. Over 600 news stories are distributed daily to ensure that cancer patients and their families have access to the most current information available in order to help them receive high-quality treatment and gain access to the newest cancer drugs and treatment strategies through the clinical trials process. Named one of the top 5 oncology Web sites by Oncology Net Guide. Endorsed by the National Patient Advocate Foundation and the Oncology Nursing Society.

CenterWatch
www.centerwatch.com
Clinical trials listing service. Provides an extensive list of approved clinical trials being conducted internationally and lists of promising therapies newly approved by the FDA (Food and Drug Administration). In-depth reports on specific illnesses, clinical trials and new medical therapies available for purchase.

Clinicaltrails.gov
www.clinicaltrails.gov
Registry of federally and privately supported clinical trials conducted in the United States and around the world. Information about a trial's purpose, who may participate, locations, and phone numbers for more details. This information should be used in conjunction with advice from health care professionals.

Dana Farber Cancer Institute – Zakim Center for Integrated Therapies
http://www.dana-farber.org
Principal teaching affiliate of Harvard Medical School, supports more than 200,000 patient visits a year involved in clinical trials. Internationally renowned expertise in bringing novel therapies that prove beneficial and safe in the laboratory setting into clinical use.

ECancerTrials.com
ecancertrials.com
Free and confidential clinical trials matching and referral services. Up-to-date information on over 2000 clinical trials in oncology. Privately search for clinical trials applicable to your situation independently or with assistance.

EnergyGrid Alternative Magazine
www.energygrid.com/health/cancer-cure.html
A regularly updated guide to point individuals in directions that could help maximize survival chances. Also provides guidance of life-style, supplementation and dietary measures to support more conventional treatments.

Federation of Chiropractic Licensing Boards
www.fclb.org/boards.htm
Find licensed chiropractors listed by state.

Gilda's Club Worldwide
www.gildasclub.org
Gilda's Clubs offer support and networking groups, seminars, workshops, specialized children's programs and social events, in a home-like setting free of charge. Offers support services to people with cancer and their family and friends.

Healing Touch Program: Leaders in Energy Medicine

www.healingtouchprogram.com

The Healing Touch Program offers a series of energy-based therapy classes in which students use a variety of hands-on techniques that facilitate energy balance for wholeness within the individual, supporting physical, emotional, mental and spiritual well being. The Healing Touch Program has been taught since 1989 to more than 96,000 participants worldwide. and include a medically-based energy therapy training program for nurses.

Health World Online

www.healthy.net

Resources in nutrition, fitness, self-care and mind/body approaches to maintaining high-level health and well-being.

Hopelab.org

www.hopelab.org

www.re-mission.net

HopeLab is exploring new ways to address chronic illness. Creators of a ground-breaking videogame, Re-Mission™, proven to help patients fight cancer. Research shows that playing Re-Mission improved treatment adherence and produced increases in quality of life, self-efficacy, and cancer-related knowledge for adolescents and young adults with cancer. Re-Mission is available free of charge at www.re-mission.net

Illuminata: A Return to Prayer by Marianne Williamson

Published Random House, Inc.

This spiritual book is a way to bring prayer into practical use, to release us from a deep and abiding psychic pain. Through prayer we find what we cannot find elsewhere: a peace that is not of this world.

International Society for Reiki Training

www.reiki.org

Reiki is a Japanese technique for stress reduction and relaxation that also promotes healing. It's administered by laying on hands and can be easily learned by anyone. This site offers information including free practice and teaching materials.

National Center for Complementary and Alternative Medicine (NCCAM)

www.nccam.nih.gov

1-888-644-6226 (Toll-Free)

Federal Government's lead agency for scientific research on complementary and alternative medicines. Sponsors and conducts research using scientific methods and advanced technologies to study diverse medical and health care systems, practices, and products that are not presently considered to be part of conventional medicine. Provides timely and accurate information about research and helps the public and health professionals understand which therapies have been proven to be safe and effective.

National Certification Board for Therapeutic Massage and Bodywork

www.ncbtmb.com

Find a nationally certified practitioner nearby. Search for a professional by name – or by the city/state/zip you're in. You can also specify the type (modality) of therapeutic massage or bodywork you prefer.

National Certification Commission for Acupuncture and Oriental Medicine (NCCAOM)

www.nccaom.org

Search for practitioners who are nationally certified in Oriental Medicine, Acupuncture, Chinese Herbology,and Asian Bodywork Therapy. Contact information provided for Individuals certified in Oriental Medicine have met requirements for board certification in both Acupuncture AND Chinese Herbology.

National Institutes of Health-Clinical Center

www.cc.nih.gov

Information on current clinical trial research and participating in clinical trials. The Clinical Center at the National Institutes of Health (NIH) in Bethesda, Maryland, is the nation's largest hospital devoted entirely to clinical research.

National Library of Medicine – Pubmed

www.pubmed.com

Medical article search tool. Includes over 17 million citations from MEDLINE and other life science journals for biomedical articles back to the 1950s. PubMed includes links to full text articles and other related resources

Natural Standard

www.naturalstandard.com

Comprehensive information on CAM therapies. Natural Standard is impartial; not supported by any interest group, professional organization, product manufacturer. Institutional subscriptions, custom content and licensing are available.

Plum Village Practice Center

www.plumvillage.org

Unified Buddhist Church, Inc.

Buddhist monastery and mindfulness practice center for monks, nuns and lay people. Founded during the Vietnam war by Thich Nhat Hanh, a Vietnamese Buddhist monk, poet, scholar, and peace activist. His life long efforts to generate peace and reconciliation moved Martin Luther King, Jr. to nominate him for the Nobel Peace Prize in 1967. When not travelling the world to teach "The Art of Mindful Living." Hanh teaches, writes, and gardens in Plum Village.

The Gleanings Foundation

www.gleaningsfoundation.org

The Gleanings Foundation explores the connections of human consciousness and universal awareness based on the concept that when a human being connects to a universal energy, all things are possible, including finding an answer to a medical problem, a message in a crisis, or just a shift in a perception.

United States Conference of Catholic Bishops

www.usccb.org

www.catholichawaii.org

Find a church and support group near you.

U.S. Food and Drug Administration (FDA)

Check for safety alerts on CAM therapies.

http://www.fda.gov/opacom/7alerts.html

Well Spouse Foundation

www.wellspouse.org

Provides social support to spouses and partners.

HAWAI'I SPECIFIC

American Cancer Society (ACS)

www.cancer.org

808-595-7500 (Hawai'i Chapter)

Find out what's going on in Hawai'i including upcoming events, news, local resources, volunteer opportunities, and more. Referrals to practical assistance with housing, medical equipment and supplies, wigs and accessories, support groups and support services and transportation.

Bosom Buddies of Hawai'i

www.bosombuddieshi.org

Offers several locations to receive Healing Touch treatments from "Bosom Buddies" practitioners. free of charge. Our clients are encouraged to receive Healing Touch treatments as often as their schedule permits, especially near treatment and procedure dates. Our clients have experienced results ranging from increased relaxation and pain relief to enhanced recovery after surgery. Supported by many local organizations including the American Cancer Society's Reach to Recovery program and the Hawai'i Affiliate of the Susan G. Komen Breast Cancer Foundation.

Consumer Health Information Service

www.hml.org

A community service of Hawai'i Medical Library.

Hawai'i Breast and Cervical Cancer Control Program (HBCCCP)

Provides screening and diagnostic services for breast and cervical cancers for women 40-64 years of age who are under-insured and need financial assistance. The program offers free services to qualifying women including cancer information and education, clinical breast examinations, mammograms, pelvic exams, and Pap tests. HBCCCP service providers:

OAHU

Kapi`olani Women's Medical Center : 808-973-3015

Kokua Kalihi Valley : 808- 848-0976

Koolauloa Health & Wellness Center in Kahuku : 808-293-9216

St. Francis HealthCare Systems of Hawai'i : 808-547-6889

The Queen's Women Center : 808-537-7555

Waimanalo Health Clinic : 808- 259-7948, Ext. 147

HAWAI`I ISLAND
Bay Clinic, Inc. : 808- 969-1427
West Hawai`i : 808- 331-2632
Hamakua HC : 808-775-7204

KAUA`I
Kaua`i Breast & Cervical Cancer Control Project : 808- 245-7767

MAUI
Hui No Ke Ola Pono: 808- 249-0104

Hawai'i Health Guide
www.hawaiihealthguide.com
Online resource is to help you make informed choices about the resources available in Hawaii .The Health Guide is divided into 10 distinct directories including Hawaiian healing techniques, health practitioners, physicians directory

Kapi'olani Women's Center (Hawai'i)
www.kapiolaniwoman.org
808-973-5967
808-535-7000 (High-Risk Program)
Offering Women's Cancer Support Groups in addition to treatment. Kapi'olani High High-Risk Breast Cancer Prevention Program offers screening and counseling aimed at preventing breast cancer and reducing risks where genetics and family history place a woman at higher risk for breast cancer. Women without insurance or minimal insurance are eligible for the program.

Pacific Cancer Foundation
808-243-2999
www.pacificcancerfoundation.com
Assists patients and their families by providing access, advocacy and information. Provides easy and effective access to various treatment options available to cancer patients. Distills vast amount of information available on cancer to a manageable educational resource for patients, families and healthcare providers. Identifies and assists in gaining access to clinical trials and research that may be appropriate for certain patients and acts as the liaison among parties involved in these trials. Serves as an advocate for patients and their families in order to ensure that they receive the utmost respect and dignity as they face the challenges of their disease.

HAWAI'I SUPPORT GROUPS

O`AHU
Kapiolani Breast Center - Healthy Living with Cancer
808-973-3044
Kapiolani Breast Center, 1st floor, 1907 South Beretania Street

Kuakini Breast Cancer Education and Support Group
808-547-9562
347 North Kuakini Street

Pali Momi Hospital - Hui Malama Kako'o
808-486-5502
Pali Momi Hospital Physician's Dining Room

Windward O`ahu Breast Cancer Support Group
808-263-5440
www.castlemed.org
Castle Medical Center Wellness Center

Women's Health Center at The Queen's Medical Center - Breast Cancer Support Group
808-585-5330
1301 Punchbowl Street

MAU`I
Mau'i Breast Cancer Support Group
808- 874-0334
Maui Adult Care Center

KAUA`I
Cancer & Lymphedema Self-Help Group
808-742-1840
808-822-3011
Borders Books & Music Maui in Lihu`e

West Hawai'i Island- (Kona and surrounding areas)
808-322-9140
Teshima's Restaurant, 79-7251 Mamalahoa Hwy, Kealakekua

East Hawai'i Island- (Hilo & surrounding areas)
808 -935-9763
Hilo Medical Center Conference Room
1190 Waianuenue Ave, Hil

CREDITS

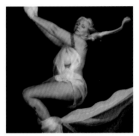

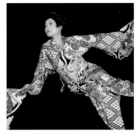

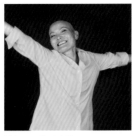

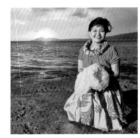

Make-up: Kecia Littman
www.keciabella.com
Make-up Asst: Carol Tagawa
Hair Stylist: Dell Taylor
Tiffany Replogo

Make-up: Wendy Robin
www.StudioWofHonolulu.com
Wardrobe : Tony Apilado
Location : Pacific Focus Inc.

Make-up: Kecia Littman
www.keciabella.com
Make-up Asst: Carol Tagawa
Hair Stylist: Dell Taylor
Tiffany Replogo

Make-up: Zairrah -
zairrah @ yahoo.com

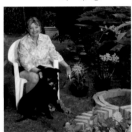

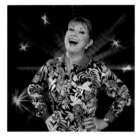

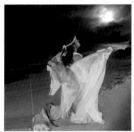

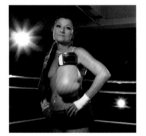

Make-up: Recyne Sugai
www.makeup808.com

Make-up: Kecia Littman -
www.keciabella.com
Location: Ohana West Studios
www.OhanaWestStudios.com

Hair: Dennis Guillermo
Make-up: Taryn Yamada
Location: Salon 808

Make-up: Kecia Littman
www.keciabella.com

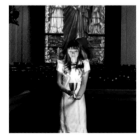

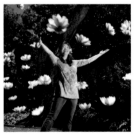

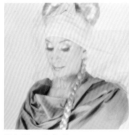

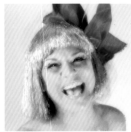

Make-up: Crystal Pancipanci -
www.pancistyle.com
Location: Cathedral of Our Lady
Of Peace

CathedralofOurLadyofPeace.com

Make-up: Biyoushi
www.biyoushihawaii.com
Location: Foster Botanical Gardens

Make-up Crystal Pancipanci -
www.pancistyle.com
Wardrobe :Tony Apilado
Location: Palolo Gym

Make-up: Madoka Tsubokawa
Location: Salon 808

Photo Assistants: Lance Holden • Wendy H. • Cynthia Ochoa • Jose Oquindo • Lynsey Rivers • Oronde Domonique

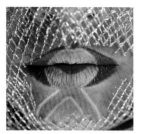

Make-up: Kecia Littman
www.keciabella.com
Make-up Asst: Carol Tagawa

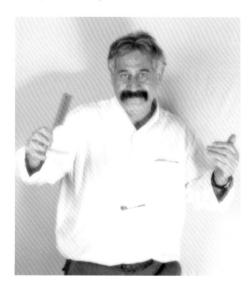

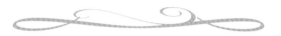

OUR HERO ~ HENRY RAMIREZ
SALON 808, HONOLULU

Henry isn't a doctor but he's helped heal thousands of breast cancer patients in the past several years. He generously donates his time and talents styling and fitting wigs, shaving heads and offering words of comfort and cheer to his customers, including many of the women in this book. Henry dedicates at least 3 appointments a day, 6 days a week to guiding cancer patients through the traumatic journey of hair loss with gentle optimisim, experienced wisdom and talent.

He says, "Cancer can be heartbreaking. I tell women that cancer marks a change in life. And as I style their hair and wigs and tell them, it won't be like it was before, but it will be beautiful. Then I do everything I can to make it so. If my skills can help someone, I'm grateful to be able to do it."

In the words of one survivor, "Henry is a prince. He made me see myself in a way I never had before. He made me see my beauty and the beauty of my life. And whenever I saw him, I always felt better. I owe him a lot."

We thank Henry for his love and compassion and for igniting the spirits of breast cancer survivors. He reminds us that we all have the power to help.

About the Photographer

PHOTGRAPHER: James Anshutz (*www.JamesAphoto.com*)

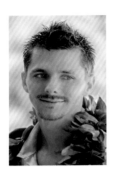

Born and raised in Tampa Florida, James ("Jay") Anshutz has been taking photos since the age of ten. At twenty three he felt a calling to move to Hawai'i despite the fact that he knew very little about it. When he stepped off the plane, he knew he had found his spiritual home. Jay later fell in love with a local girl, married her and started his family. Inspired by the spirit of the islands and a chance meeting with a stranger who purchased his first artistic photo, James made the leap from hobbiyst to professional photograper. He continues to hone his craft.

Aside from his family and friends, Jay's greatest love is collaborating with a creative team on his shoots to promote consciousness of social issues. As a youth, Jay worked with his mother as a volunteer helping in nursing homes and working with HIV-positive children. He continues his working with at-risk youth and autistic children. His goal is to open a community center for the arts and music for at-risk youth and disabled individuals and to create more books. His whimsical and dramatic style has captured the attention of our local fashion and commercial photography industry. This is Jay's first book. You can see more of Jay's work at jamesaphoto.com.

Photographer's Special Thanks

First and foremost...God, Buddha, The Universe, or whatever word you would choose for the spirit.

To my mom and dad, Lorrie and Dave, for all of their love, financial support, and raising me to think of others and strive to be a better person. To my wife Cara for her motivation, patience, amazing ideas, love, and support throughout this project. It would not be possible if it wasn't for YOU. To my kids Koa and Bodhi for their patience for daddy/uncle having to always go to work. To my spiritual teacher Craig for his guidance and meditations, and all of our world's spiritual leaders and spirits for assisting us through life and transformations. To my biological mom, Lee, for giving birth to me and having the courage to do what she did. To my Grandpa for putting me in touch with Lee and being an inspiration even though I didn't get to know him very well on this physical plane. To my brothers Chad and Donny, & kinda step dad Dave. To all my mainland family and friends: Cuzin Gus, Brandi, Lauren, Scott, Aunt Carol, Uncle Glen, Sean J. and Saisha J., Jamie J., Ramona J. (another mom), Uncle John J, Izzy and Dylan, Nate Dogg, Rosie, Skylar, Wendy, the Grattans, Amber E. and Dan B., Ivyia T. and Fam, Aaron and Cristy Button, oh and Bosco, Cameron, Adrianna, Taylor and all my Tampa folks. Ritalin.

To Hawai'i: Mahalo nã akua, nã 'aumakua, a me Ko'u 'ohana a pau.

To the Hawai'i folks: All of the wonderful women and children that participated in this project, to their familys for their support throughout the journey of this process. Tony Apilado for his amazing creativity, art direction, and emotional support!! Marie and Kurt Winner for all of their help and referrals...this project wouldn't have gotten off the ground if it wasn't for you. To the Cathedral staff and volunteers. To JoDee and Ernie for their support and gallery space. All of the wonderful teams of MUA's, Stylists, Assistants, and behind the scenes staff listed above that made this thing happen and look fabulous. Straub Hospital and Kapi'olani Women's Center Oncology Dept. Specifically: Claire T., Brigette, & Suzanne D. Henry and Jaime at Salon 808 and their wonderful and amazing hairstylists and make-up artists. The program folks. All of our friends, family. Stephanie, Bert, Felise, Francesco, Dwight and Kay O., John Woodward aka "Richard", Kathleen at On Board 4 A Cure, Ken W., Sean, Danny and Victoria L., CeCe Akim, aka "Puna", Corrine and family, Darren and Family. To all of the PPH and PPA people, and the people we come in contact with that change our lives forever especially the woman who bought my first photographic art while printing it at Kinko's... Thank you. To anyone I may have forgotten or didn't have room to list (you do realize this is a coffee table book)... Thank you from the bottom of my heart.

To those who helped bring the first show to life: Jake and Jeff of Artist Island (www.artistisland.com) for their print service donations, King Photo (Honolulu) for saving my butt with thier emergency print services and product donations. Brian Bilberry and PPA for legal guidance and support. PPH for moral support. Save The Tatas for their product donation and sponsorship. Injoy Marketing & O'ahu Computer Consulting for website development. Lance Holden of Holden Graphic Design for logo and graphic design. Pictures on tile by John Hillcrest. Chad Tarbutton for his art and graphic contributions(www.NotJustAwall.com). Chinatown Courtyard (Honolulu) - JoDee and Ernie from First Friday Artwalk (www.firstfridayhawaii.com). Bill & Liz Labbey donated studio time for the shoot and the Honolulu Film Office. And finally to Aloun Farms for letting me get lost in thier corn field.

~ Jay

About the Author

AUTHOR & DESIGNER: Cynthia Y.H. Derosier

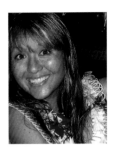 Born and raised in Hawai'i, Cynthia left for New York City to earn her BFA in Art Direction and Design and went on to work as an Art Director and Creative Director at several prestigious agencies. She returned home over a decade later, wanting to work on more personal and meaningful projects and give back to Hawai'i and her community.

In 2005, Cynthia woke up from a restless sleep and realized she had dreamt a book. She was not a writer and had no experience in publishing, but her instincts told her that producing the book would be a good thing for her community and would somehow help others. With the support of family and friends *The Surfer Spirit* was born.

The Surfer Spirit was brought to life by Cynthia and a *hui* ~ a cooperative team ~ of surfers, a minister, a lama and an esteemed Hawaiian Kumu and reflects how surfing is a metaphor for life. Surfing is not just a sport, or even a "lifestyle." The need to surf goes beyond trends, fashion, ego, competition and camaraderie. It's the way surfers experience the essential spirit of life. This zen-like book features stunning photos with simple profound sentiments that inspire surfers and non-surfers alike.

Today the book has become a local best-seller and is making waves in the corporate and the non-profit world. It's the basis for a program that helps at-risk youth live better lives through surfing and an other that is helping businesses build stronger teams and inspire their staff.

She has become a passionate promoter of "The Good Juju", reminding us to reconnect to life by celebrating our joys and honoring and nourishing our spirits. *The Survivor Spirit* is Cynthia's second book in The Spirit Series by Free Time Productions | The Good Juju Co. Two more books are due for release at the end of 2009. A portion of the sale of each book goes to support related non-profit programs in our community.

www.goodjujuco.com

Author's Special Thanks

Great teams of great people make works for the greater good possible.
My heartfelt gratitude goes out to those who helped me keep the spirit alive and be as pono as possible.
My very special thanks to Kahu and Sharon Silva for your blessings and guidance ~ you helped me
see the path more clearly so I could walk it confidently. To Ramsay Taum for the light of his work and
for joining me on this journey. To the Lovitts for thier open hearts and support that made the dream
a reality and enabled the good juju to grow. To Seth Reiss and Flip McCuddy for helping me keep the
spirit alive and guiding me safely through the fire. To Casey, Sheri, Annabel, and Ruth for riding the
rough seas with me when no one else would. To Makana and Sundae for your wisdom, assistance and
the inspirations of our hui. To Mel for your sharp vision! To Tim Anderson and Jim Elder for their
talents and contributions. To Jane, Myra, Anna Marie, Sharon and all the women who shared thier
stories. To Bev Motz and David Reno for nurturing this baby and the one before it. And especially to
my mother, my grandfather, my monk great uncle, and all my ancestors, who taught me to believe in
my spirit and follow inspiriation.

Share the Good Juju!

Our books are dedicated to promoting the positive spirit. *The Surfer Spirit* has been
changing lives through the Spirit Sessions. A portion of each sale of *The Survivor Spirit*
goes to non-profit programs supporting breast cancer awareness and the search for a cure.

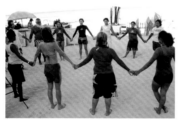

Sessions start with a quick talk circle
and yoga warm-up.

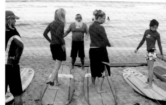

Teens get a beach lession from surf
instructors before hitting the water.

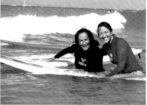

The Girls Court therapist and surf
mentors cheer for the girls in and
out of the water.

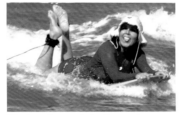

Mentors demonstrate the most
important part of life and surfing.
Work hard and have fun!

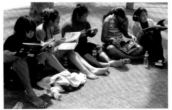

The teens comtemplate life lessons
found in the book and in the water
and record them in journals.

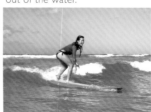

Catching waves and changing lives,
the Spirit Sessions is working!